ALL YOU WANTED TO KNOW ABOUT
Jnana Yoga

SWAMI ATMANANDA
(Prof. Ravindra Kumar PhD)

New Dawn

NEW DAWN
An imprint of Sterling Publishers (P) Ltd.
A-59 Okhla Industrial Area, Phase-II,
New Delhi-110020.
Tel: 6313023, 6320118, 6916165, 6916209
Fax: 91-11-6331241 E-mail: ghai@nde.vsnl.net.in
www.sterlingpublishers.com

All you wanted to know about Jnana Yoga
© 2002, Sterling Publishers Private Limited
ISBN 81 207 2434 8

Published by Sterling Publishers Pvt. Ltd., New Delhi-110020.
Lasertypeset by Vikas Compographics, New Delhi-110020.
Printed at Sai Printers, New Delhi-110020.

Contents

Contents

Preface

Jnana yoga is the 'path of knowledge'. It was designed in the vedic period, for people with stronger minds than the hearts. It is basically the method of finding an answer to the question, 'Who am I?' One keeps pondering on all possible answers and goes on negating them one by one, till the right answer is reached. The right answer is that one is soul or *atma*, and since *atma* is akin to God, one gets an intuitive understanding of God. Notable *jnanayogis* were King Janaka, Socrates, etc.

Although Jnana yoga is in itself the complete path to the knowledge of self and God, the right approach would be to first undergo Karma yoga to achieve equanimity and an equipoise mind, and then undergo Jnana yoga to know first hand that there exists a superintelligence called God, and finally to undergo Bhakti yoga to taste the Godhood personally. Without the taste of God in person, dry philosophical knowledge does not give full satisfaction; one keeps missing something – joy or bliss.

This book presents the elements of Jnana yoga in a simple and comprehensive way, so that it is understandable to the common man. Simple and practical methods are presented that have been followed at the Academy of Kundalini Yoga and Quantum Soul (AKYQS) for a long time. The publisher deserves congratulations for his attempts to present the truth to the general masses. I wish to thank William Henry Belk II for his support and encouragement. Sincere thanks are due to Jytte Kumar Larsen for the many thought-provoking discussions and for computing help and facilities.

Swami Atmananda (Ravindra Kumar PhD)
Founder President, Academy of Kundalini
Yoga and Quantum Soul.
58-61 Vashisht Park, Pankha Road, New
Delhi-110046
Tel: 504 7091, 504 7089
E-mail: ravijytte@now-india.net.in
And,
Sofus Francks Vaenge 6,6
DK 2000, Frederiksberg, Denmark
Tel: (45) 36 16 92 50
Email: JytteRavi.Kumar@mail.tele.dk

Introduction

Though the path of knowledge, which is Jnana yoga, is enough to bring self/God realisation, yet the natural sequence is *karma, jnana* and *bhakti*, in that very order. Karma yoga is the path of selfless action in which one acts without expecting the fruits of one's actions. When this is successful, the practitioner achieves an equipoise mind. With this mind the practitioner then follows Jnana yoga, which ultimately leads him/her to the knowledge of the Supreme Being or God. After this, it is Bhakti yoga, the path of devotion, which unites the person with God Almighty. Karma yoga should be of the order of Mahatma Gandhi or Mother Teresa, and Jnana yoga should be of the order of Socrates and Ramana Maharishi, before you can expect some results. However, if you combine the three paths simultaneously, you have greater chances of success in a single lifetime, with fewer obstacles on the way.

Unless *bhakti* (devotion) is practised, *karma* and *jnana* will lead to dry knowledge, which does not give full satisfaction. You miss the *rasa* (joy) which comes only through devotion, which induces love; and love is God. This is the importance of devotion, which has also been emphasised by Lord Krishna. It is based on the practice followed at the centres of Academy of Kundalini Yoga and Quantum Soul.

Creation and Properties of the Soul

According to the Oxford dictionary the soul is the non-material part of a person, believed to exist forever; whereas according to the Webster's it is an entity without material reality, considered to be the spiritual part of a person. Putting these definitions together we can say that, the soul is the non-material and spiritual part of a person, that exists forever.

The *Bhagavad Gita* (Prabhupad, 1968) records the teachings of Lord

Krishna, spoken several millennia ago, with the following substance. For the soul there is neither birth nor death at any time. It has not come into being; it does not come into being; and it will not come into being. It is unborn, eternal, ever-existing and primeval. It is not slain when the body is slain. The embodied soul continuously passes through the different stages of a person, from childhood to youth to old age, it similarly passes into another body at death. Those who have realised the truth have concluded that the non-existent (the material body) does not endure and the eternal (soul) does

13

not change. This they have concluded by studying the nature of both. No one is able to destroy the imperishable soul. Just as a person dons a new garment, giving up an old one, similarly, the soul accepts new material bodies, giving up the old and useless ones. The soul can never be cut into pieces by any weapon, nor burned by fire, or moistened by water, or withered by the wind. The individual soul is unbreakable and insoluble. It is everlasting, present everywhere, unchangeable, immovable and eternally the same. It is said that the soul is invisible, inconceivable and immutable. Knowing this, you should not grieve for the body. All created beings are unmanifest in their beginning, manifest in their interim state, and unmanifest again when annihilated. So what need is there for lamentation?

It is believed that it was not for the first time that the *Bhagavad Gita* was explained by Lord Krishna in the battlefield of Kurukshetra some five thousand years ago. It was on the planet sun, some tens of thousand years ago, that sage Manu had taught the principles of the *Bhagavad Gita*. And later at some future date the same principles will be taught again.

15

Aldous Huxley called it 'perennial philosophy' (Huxley, 1944).

And now the psychics, and past-life-regressionists are independently discovering the same principles. More details about the physics of the soul are coming up. Souls are found to be made of energy, they are beings of light, they can take on any shape they want—sometimes appearing in human form, sometimes as streaks of light or blobs of energy. Whatever the form, it is totally alive energy, which is thinking and feeling, being with memories or unresolved issues, and possessing a sense of humour. (Bodine, 1999). The soul is mightier than space, stronger than time, deeper than the sea, and higher than the stars. While the soul is out-of-the-body, the perceptions suddenly get highly intensified, (for example, the crying of a child in the neighbouring room becomes clearer and louder [Wilson, 1987]).

The travelling of the soul is an important aspect, which needs attention. The soul is connected with the body through a silver cord which can stretch to an unlimited length when it travels out of the body. The cord is severed only at the time of physical death. It is the conscious mind, which governs the journey of the soul, either out of the body or back into the body. Although major soul-travel experiences take place during sleep, the soul also goes out for small trips during waking hours, although we do not·consciously know about it. Some of the symptoms, which indicate a possible out-of-the-body experience of the soul during sleep, are as follows:

- Most of the flying dreams appear to be real.
- Dreams of visiting the deceased, or loved ones appear to be real.
- Dreams of being close to a loved one living in a faraway place, with a sad feeling of a forced separation on waking up.

- Sometimes you wake up in the middle of the night but you can neither open your eyes nor move your body, nor can you open your mouth to tell someone about it.
- You are shaken for a second in the middle of the night, but you go to sleep again after a momentary waking up.

There are moments when the soul goes out of the body for brief periods during waking hours. It happens during intense emotional feelings, such as concern for a loved one who is sick, or desire of being with a loved one who is far away, or seeing a cherished part of the world which you cannot visit physically, or concern for your children or for some work in progress in another part of the city. One feels like day-dreaming or going blank during such periods of absence of the soul from the body. During such periods you may kiss or hug a person briefly, and the person will not know it consciously but will have a feeling of being loved. Many times you may feel that someone is calling you by your name; in fact, a soul is actually around and calling you, but the physical senses do not have the capacity of sensing it. Amnesia creates a barrier to the conscious mind, so that the mind cannot know everything the soul knows. That is why when the soul goes out briefly, the mind goes blank. The soul has visited the loved one, but the conscious mind does not know about it. The soul uses the body and the mind for the experiences of the current incarnation. The body and mind are limited within the five senses but the soul is not.

There are some other situations during which the soul travels. If you go to bed with some unsolved problems on your mind, the soul may go out of the body and talk to other souls to find the solution, and you wake up with an answer in the morning. You do not consciously know the homework done by the soul, but you are happy at the discovery. When physically unable to take a vacation, the soul may travel out of the body when it is asleep, visit the place of interest, such as a garden or a hill station, for quite some time. You wake up refreshed with a smile in the morning, not knowing again the homework done by the soul. Sometimes you see the whole experience as a dream, and feel happy about having dreamt of the place of your liking. Yet the reason of happiness is the soul-travel. In the case of an abuse, the soul may leave the body at the start, and return when it is over. For a few months before and after birth, the soul is known to go out and re-enter the body, as many times as it likes. The same thing happens when you are in the process of dying – the soul goes out of the body, sometimes for completing an unfinished task, or sometimes for preparing a home in the other world.

Although soul-travel dreams occur spontaneously, some people learn how to induce them. And again, although the state of sleep is conducive to the experience, it is not necessary to sleep to have an out-of-body-experience. Terrill Wilson (1987) could consciously come out of his body after about a year's practice of concentration. He used to focus his attention at a distant place, feel the smell of the room, think about the history of things in there, etc. For several years he travelled from one layer to another and interacted with many people on the way. He has prescribed improved formulas for coming out of the body. However, in the end, he says that it is spiritual perfection and not soul-travel which should be our aim.

Robert A. Monroe has established an institution for soul-travel in the

United States, after writing several books on out-of-body experiences. There are three techniques that can be used for the purpose. First is the technique of 'mind awake and body asleep', in which one tries to remain conscious when the body goes to sleep. Slowly one enters the twilight zone, which is the middle state between sleeping and waking, and then one can think of becoming lighter and lighter, and finally rising up and moving away. Either one feels the sensation of moving out through the top of the head or one suddenly finds oneself in the subtle body. Second is the technique of 'rotation', in which one attempts to turn over without using the arms and legs for help, while in the twilight zone. After a 180 degree turn, one should think of floating up and away from the body. Third is the technique of 'sexual energy', in which one arouses one's passions and then sublimates the energy instead of releasing it physically. One should imagine the energy as a white globe, rising from the root centre (*mooladhar chakra*) to the eyebrow centre (*ajna chakra*) or the crown centre (*sahasrar*), and then rising up and away from the body. Some people feel a roaring or buzzing sensation while going out-of-body, like the vibrations of a motor when you start it. There are different experiences with different people while undergoing soul-travel.

Although the time of creation of the souls cannot be traced back, some believe that it was around ten billion years ago. However, we all hear about references to old souls and new souls, which means that old souls are the ones who have lived many lifetimes and have gained wisdom in the process, while the new ones have not yet lived many lives. Old souls move very fast out of their bodies towards their home in the heavens, average souls do not move so rapidly, while younger souls remain attached to the earth's environment right after death (Newton, 1994). Souls in a high state of advancement are often found in humble circumstances on earth. Those living in a highly influential society are not in a blissful state of soul maturity. Advanced souls do not feel lonely. Richness of diversity and the capacity to be alone is a measure of emotional and spiritual maturity. All this may suggest that the creation of souls has been taking place at different times or that God has been creating souls continually.

A past life regressionist (Newton, 2000) has taken a number of people out of their bodies under hypnosis, and has collected information about the creation of souls. There exists a sort of 'soul nursery' as reported by some newly born younger souls, and also by some incubator mothers who help in hatching the eggs and looking after the newly born souls. The nursery is a vast emporium with unlimited outside dimensions, gaslike, with swirling currents of energy above an intense light. The new souls stay in their incubator cells until they are grown enough to be taken out of the emporium. New souls are small masses of white energy encased in gold sacs moving majestically on orchestrated lines of progression. Incubator mothers in their delivery suits receive them and nurture them. The origin of production is a molten mass of high-intensity, energy and vitality, which is energised by some amazing love force rather than some heat source. The mass has the colour of the inside of eyelids and pulsates and undulates. A swelling begins in the mass, it increases, pushes outwards and separates as a new soul, alive with energy and a distinctness. Beyond the mass one can see the beatific glow of orange-yellow, and violet-darkness.

The incubator mothers hover around the hatching so that they can towel-dry them after opening the gold sacs. It is like hugging the new white energy, with blue and violet glowing around them. It is like a string of pearls moving on a silvery conveyer belt. There comes a life force of all-knowing love, and knowledge and awakening takes place in the soul through the touch of the mother. Each soul has unique characteristics which cannot be described. No two souls are alike. In other words, the source is like a divine mother who would never create twin children. The creator appears to be around but unrecognisable and perhaps assisted by others.

The purpose of creation of the world and the souls is to develop us and the world to the highest possible potential. An unlimited number of lifetimes have been given to each soul to learn in the earth-school, away from its true home where it belongs. Perfection already exists in the heavens, but each soul has to reach that stage of perfection individually. This needs going through a large variety of down-to-earth-experiences and learning everything first hand, until godhood is achieved.

It is hard for science and even for laymen like us to believe the reality of the spiritual world since the phenomena there "exist outside the electromagnetic spectrum that defines what science uses to characterise our physical world" (Gough and Shaklett, 2000). Nevertheless, individual scientists keep trying to bridge the gap between science and the spiritual world. Modern researchers have used electronic instruments to show that "individuals on the astral plane have a body composed of finer matter and vibrations. There is no sickness, and sexual intercourse

33

exists without pregnancy. Their thoughts create their reality and they communicate telepathically. One's personality is unchanged from what it was on earth, yet intellectual growth continues. One's mind determines the body's appearance, limbs that one may have lost while on earth, are once more with the body, disfigurations become perfect and the age one appears to be is subject to choice, usually between 25 to 30. By the powers of thought, one can wipe away hunger pangs. The astral plane is considered an interim place where one either reincarnates back to physical earth, moves to another planet, or moves to a higher level or plane" (Kumar, 2001).

A person who realises that he/she is a soul or *atma* has graduated from the school of earth, and the chain of death and rebirth is broken for him/her once and for all. It is one's choice now, whether he/she wants to incarnate again for the sake of teaching others, or wants to proceed further on to higher realms to get closer to God. There is always one more step on the ladder of spiritual perfection.

Fundamentals of Jnana Yoga

The path of knowledge is perhaps in prominence at present since it includes the 'official science', which is in search of 'truth' in its own experimental way, and the 'western approach', which is mainly the intellectual search for truth. This also includes the parapsychological and psychic search, for example, the work of Jung and others. Yet, the recognition of the potentialities of the human intellect by *Vedanta* will leave the people aghast at their own incapacity to make complete use of their intellect in the search for truth. *Vedanta* travels the path of pure reason and inculcates in us the jewel of discrimination between what is false and true in us; between the permanent and temporal; between the real and unreal; and leads us to self-discovery, to the knowledge that self and God are one by identity. This is the glory of Hinduism. This path has also been called *raja yoga*, (the king of yogas). King Janaka, father-in-law of Lord Rama, was perhaps the first recognised *rajayogi*.

Ramana Maharishi used to ponder all the time only on one question - who am I? And one day he arrived at the realisation that *atma* and Brahman are identical. Sankaracharya, Vivekananda, Socrates, Aristotle, Plato, Gurdjief, Steiner, William Wordsworth, Richard Maurice Bucke, etc. were all thinkers belonging to the category of a *rajayogi*. Of course, there may be variations in their stages of perfection. The progression of steps is more or less the same as in Karma yoga, and, of course, the final realisation too is the same. One goes on removing cover after cover of ignorance, just like removing the sheaths of a cabbage or onion one-by-one, and finally reaching the goal one day. Beginning with the *Vedantas*, vast literature is available, both in the East and the West. For example, Swami Vivekananda has written fifteen volumes of nearly five hundred pages each on the subject.

The fact is that knowledge takes the individual to a certain stage of development or evolution; and then the mind ceases to exist, and wisdom takes over, which is a direct perception of truth from beyond. The following observations should prove enlightening. I begin with Sri Aurobindo.

***

- Late, I learned that when reason died wisdom was born; before that liberation, I had only knowledge.

There are two allied powers in man: knowledge and wisdom. Knowledge is so much of the truth, seen in a distorted medium, as the mind arrives at after groping; wisdom is what the eye of the divine vision sees in the spirit.

When I speak, reason says, 'This will I say'; but God takes the words from my mouth and my lips say something else, at which reason trembles.

If mankind could see, though in a glimpse of fleeting experience, what the infinite enjoyments, the perfect forces, the luminous reaches of spontaneous knowledge are, what wide calms of our being lie waiting for using the tracts which our animal evolution has not yet conquered, they would leave all and never rest till they have gained these treasures. But the way is narrow, the doors are hard to force, and fear, distrust and skepticism are there. The sentinels of nature forbid the turning away of our feet from her ordinary pastures.

Reason divides, fixes details and contrasts them; wisdom unifies and marries contrasts in a single harmony.

What the soul sees and has experienced, that it knows; the rest is appearance, prejudice and opinion.

Immortality is not the survival of the mental personality after death, (though that also is true) but the waking possession of the unborn and deathless self, of which body is only an instrument and a shadow.

They proved to me convincingly that God did not exist, and I believed them. Afterwards I saw God, for He came and embraced me. And now, what should I believe, the reasoning of others or my own experience?

Hallucination is the term of science for those irregular glimpses we have of truths shut out from us by our preoccupation with matter. That which men term as hallucination is the reflection in the mind and senses of that which is beyond our ordinary mental and sensory perceptions.

Logic is the worst enemy of truth, as self-righteousness is the worst enemy of virtue; for the one cannot see its own errors nor the other its own imperfections.

The sign of dawning knowledge is to feel that as yet I know little or nothing; and yet, if I could only know my knowledge, I already possess everything.

When wisdom comes, her first lesson is, 'There is no such thing as knowledge; there are only apaches of the Infinite Deity.'

If men took life less seriously, they could very soon make it more perfect. God never takes his work seriously; therefore one looks out on this wonderful universe.

Knowledge is a child—with its achievements, it runs about the streets whooping and shouting.

Wisdom conceals her achievements for a long time in a thoughtful and mighty silence.

The love of solitude is a sign of the disposition towards knowledge; but knowledge itself is only achieved when we have a settled perception of solitude in the crowd, in the battle and in the mart.

- The supernatural is that the nature of which we have not yet attained or do not yet know, or the means of which we have not yet conquered. The common taste for miracles is the sign that man's ascent is not yet finished.

- Revelation is the direct sight, the direct hearing or the inspired memory of truth, *drishti*, *shruti*, *smriti*. It is the highest experience and always accessible to renewed experience. Not because God spoke it, but because the soul saw it. It is the word of the scriptures, our supreme authority.

- All disease is a means towards some new joy of health, all evil and pain a tuning of nature, for some more intense bliss and good, all death an opening on widest immortality. Why and how this should be so is God's secret, which only the soul purified of egoism can penetrate.

In God's providence there is no evil; but only good or its preparation.

• Religion and philosophy seek to rescue man from his ego; then the kingdom of heaven within, will be spontaneously reflected in an external divine city.

Comments

• Reason and knowledge takes one to a certain stage, after which spontaneous knowledge and wisdom takes over, leading to experiences of the soul which are permanent. One experiences God directly, and one has the conscious knowledge of the permanent self. Reflection in the mind and senses of that which is beyond our ordinary mental and sensory perceptions is called hallucination by science. Supernatural is that the means of which have not yet been conquered. Revelation is the direct experience of the soul, not something which God says.

- It is in solitude that the spirit talks to the practitioner and one has spiritual experiences. True solitude exists even in a crowd or a battlefield, and it is the measure of emotional maturity. One should tread the unfrequented ways, as Master Pythagoras said, and develop love of solitude. In this manner one can open oneself to God.

***

There are two for whom there is hope, the man who has felt God's touch and been drawn to it and the skeptical seeker and self-convinced atheist; but for the formulariser of all the religions and the parrots of free thoughts, they are dead souls who follow a death that they call living.

Comments

Sri Aurobindo points out two possible ways of approaching God: (i) With faith, surrender and devotion to God one is drawn closer to Him and one experiences God one day in various ways (ii) A skeptical seeker who questions everything and keeps asking the question 'who am I', reaches the 'truth' one day. The former is the path of devotion and the latter is the path of knowledge. One has to choose the path of his or her liking and go deep into it. Others who are in-between, cannot master the process either way, and they cannot reach the goal of self or god-realisation.

***

If when thou art doing great actions and moving giant results, thou canst perceive that thou art doing nothing, then know that God has removed His seal from thy eyelids.

Comments

In most of the faiths and traditions it is stated that God is the only doer. Sri Aurobindo points out that the practitioner who has realised this fact and considers himself or herself as doing nothing, even when he or she may be doing works of great importance, has mastered his or her ego and is open to God now. One can understand this through a simple example. While travelling in a train one may erroneously think that it is he or she that is carrying the briefcase in hand; it is the train in fact which is carrying the briefcase. One erroneously takes the doership on himself or herself and is thus bound by *karma*. Any activity or happening which takes place is not the result of a single factor. It is the whole machinery which makes a thing happen and doership cannot be ascribed to any single factor. A car runs because it has wheels, there is gas in it, there is a driver at the steering and so on. If any single factor, such as the gas, for example, says that the car is running because of it, would be wrong. Similarly, in daily life events take place because of many known and unknown factors and any human being should not ascribe doership to himself or herself, and should leave it to nature or God. One who can do this is free of *karma* and open to God.

***

Pain is the touch of our Mother teaching us how to bear and grow in rapture. She has three stages of her schooling: endurance, equality of soul and ecstasy.

Comments

Pain and suffering is something which concerns most of us, some time or the other. An average person begins to blame God or a person or a particular circumstance for it, and wants to come out of it as early as possible. Sri Aurobindo points out that pain is caused by a divine source for teaching certain lessons which are necessary for spiritual growth. If pain is taken with patience and tolerance, and if one keeps oneself open to the divine teaching coming through it, one finally enjoys ecstasy.

***

Only by perfect renunciation of desire or by perfect satisfaction of desire can the utter embrace of God be experienced, for in both ways the essential precondition is effected — the desire perishes.

Comments

Desire perishes either by perfect renunciation or by perfect satisfaction, which is a prerequisite to the experience of God. This is the basic and perhaps the most important point on which two schools of Hindu philosophy are based. There have been *yogis* like King Harish Chandra, who controlled all his passions and renunciated all his desires. He left the throne and lived a very ordinary life. He came to beg from his own wife one day, and addressed her as '*mata*' (mother). All women for him were the form of mother; that is, complete victory over sex. One day he desired to eat some tasty pudding and laboured hard to earn the money needed for it during the day. He bought the pudding but soon after tasting it he realised that he was giving in to nature. He felt very sorry, spat out all he had in the mouth, and instead pushed cow-dung into his mouth. This is renunciation.

The other way is to satisfy all desires and come out of them realising their futility, which is the way shown by 'tantra', for example. The aspirant of God has to choose one of the two ways. Kundalini is awakened by either of the two extremities. Just as water must boil to 100 degrees to be converted into steam, so too man when he goes through practices like yoga and meditation, his human weaknesses like greed, lust, anger and attachment are converted into virtues like tolerance, compassion and humanitarian service, and gradually he is converted into God. Hence each one of us has to choose one of the two alternatives and train our lives to achieve that goal.

***

What was Ramakrishna? God manifest in a human being; but behind there is God in His infinite personality and His universal personality. And what was Vivekananda? A radiant glance from the eye of Shiva; but behind him is the Divine gaze from which he came and Shiva Himself and *Brahma* and Vishnu and 'Om' all-exceeding.

- The double law of sin and virtue is imposed on us because we have not that ideal life and knowledge within, which guides the soul spontaneously and infallibly to its self-fulfilment.

***

A saint or an *avatar* may be taken as a physical manifestation of God, yet, God Absolute is the unmanifested Infinite Being behind the personality of the saint or *avatar*, who should be the actual centre of concentration and understanding as the final goal. It is the word "om" which represents God unmanifested.

Sin and virtue exist only until the truth of soul is dormant; when self-realisation takes place, the duality of sin and virtue vanishes. There is no sin or virtue for the liberated one.

***

- Mohammed's mission was necessary, else we might have ended by thinking, in the exaggeration of our efforts at self-purification, that earth was meant only for the monk and the city created as a vestibule for the desert.

Comments

- Mohammed lived a rich and full life, marrying several times and enjoying everything. This is a pointer to the practitioners that it is not necessary to live the life of a recluse to become a saint. Even though living a full life outwardly, a person may be a real inner renunciate who is performing all physical activities in a detached way. King Janaka of Hindu mythology lived a full life with all kinds of pleasures. Once a *sadhu* (renunciate) came to stay with him. One morning they went for a walk. A celestial guru wanted to test them. He created *maya* (illusion) in which the whole palace appeared to be in flames.

King Janaka was unmoved when he saw this and said that he did not bring anything into the world and that he was not worried about their destruction. But the *sadhu* exclaimed that his *langot* (underwear) and *kamandal* (begging bowl) would get burned, and he ran towards the palace to save the two. So, who was the real renunciate? Of course the king and not the *sadhu*. The practitioner, therefore, should cultivate inner renunciation. How one lives outwardly does not really matter.

A Truly Religious Person

Various saints have talked on who a "truly religious person" is. It is interesting to note the unanimity of their views.

- Live within; be not shaken by outward happenings.

- *Sanyas* (renunciation) has a formal garb and outer tokens; therefore men think they can easily recognise it; but the freedom of a Janaka (father-in-law of Lord Rama) does not proclaim itself and it wears the garb of the world; to its presence even Narada (great sage) was blinded... Unless thou canst see the soul, how shalt thou say that a man is free or bound?

(Sri Aurobindo)

• It is not by shaving the head that one becomes a man of religion; truth and rectitude alone make the truly religious man.

(Dhammapada)

• Think not that to seat thyself in gloomy forests, in a proud seclusion, aloof from men; think not that to live on roots and plants and quench thy thirst with the snow will lead thee to the goal of the final deliverance.

(Book of the Golden Precepts)

- Though the body be adorned with jewels, the heart may have mastered worldly tendencies; he who receives with indifference joy and pain is in possession of the spiritual life even though his external existence be of the world; nor is the garb of the ascetic a protection against sensual thoughts.

    (Fo-Shu-Hing-Tsan-King)

- Although the body may be robed with the garb of the layman, the soul can raise itself to the highest perfection. The man of the world and the ascetic differ not at all from the other if both have conquered egoism. So long as the heart is bound by sensual chains, all external signs of asceticism are a vanity.

(Fo-Shu-Hing-Tsan-King)

• A solitary man may miss his goal and a man of the world become a sage.

(Fo-Shu-Hing-Tsan-King)

• A man who spreads gladness around him is better than the devotee who fasts all the year round. Fasting is a merit in the man who distributes his good to the needy; otherwise what mortification is it to take in the evening a meal you have abstained from during the day?

(Saadi)

• To take neither wine nor meat is to fast ceremonially, it is not the heart's fasting which is to maintain in oneself the one thought.

(Chuang Tse)

• And this shall be the true manner of thy fasting that thou shall be void of all iniquity.

(The Pastor of Hermes)

• It is not eating meat that makes a man impure; it is anger, intemperance, egoism, hypocrisy, disloyalty, envy, ostentation,

67

vanity and pride. It is to take pleasure in the society of those who perpetrate injustice.

(*Amaghanda Sutta*)

- Neither abstinence from meat and fish, nor mendicancy, nor shaven head or matted locks, nor mortifications of the body or garments of a special colour can purify the man who is still prey to illusion.

(Pali Canon)

- He whose mind is utterly pure from all evil as the sun is pure of stain and the moon of soil, him indeed I call a man of religion.

(Udanavagga)

- He who practises wisdom without anger or covetousness, who fulfils with fidelity his vows and is master of himself, he is indeed a man of religion.

  (Buddhist Text)

- He who watches over his body, his speech, his whole self, who is full of serenity and joy, possesses a spirit unified and finds satisfaction in solitude, he is indeed a man of religion.

  (Buddhist Text)

- He who punishes not, kills not, permits not to be killed, who is full of love among those who are full of cruelty, he is indeed a man of religion.

(Buddhist Text)

• He who has conquered the desire of present life and of the future life, who has vanquished all fear and broken all chains, he is indeed a man of religion.

(Buddhist Text)

Comments

It is not the outer appearance and outer life, but the inner attitude and inner life of a person that matters. A person may or may not be a vegetarian, he may or may not be a householder, he may be living in a

70

forest or a palace, he may have shaved his head and be wearing saffron coloured clothes, or he may have beautiful hair, wear a suit and tie, or be walking or driving a car and so on; it does not really matter. If he or she has conquered ego and pride, neither kills nor allows others to kill, is humble and compassionate to all, receives joy and pain equally, is not bound by sensual chains, practises wisdom without anger and covetousness, is full of serenity and joy, and finds satisfaction in solitude, then he or she is a religious person. Such a person may be living a full worldly life, yet he or she is close to reality and God. Another person without these virtues may be living in a monastery with shaven head and saffron coloured clothes, yet he or she is millions of miles away from the truth and God. Hence a person should devote his or her life for inner renunciation and not care for outer garb. One should aim at becoming a *yogi*, who is concerned with renunciation and not a pundit, who is theoretically knowledgeable. Of course, an ideal person is a *yogi* and a pundit put together.

Identity of the Soul and God

It is so pleasant and heartening to see that saints all over the world have been teaching one and the same thing — the identity of the soul and God. What follows are the quotations from various saints which confirm this.

- The *Vedanta* says, "Man, thou art of one nature and substance with God, one soul with thy fellowmen. Awake and progress then to the utter divinity, live for God in thyself and in others." This gospel which was given only to the few, must now be offered to all mankind for its deliverance.

Sri Aurobindo

- Why should man go about seeking God? God is in his heartbeats and he knows it not; he is wrong in seeking Him outside himself.

  God is my inmost self, the reality of my being.

  Vivekananda

- He who finds not the Eternal in himself, will never find it outside; but he who sees Him in the temple of his own soul, sees Him also in the temple of the universe.

- The individual 'I' and the Supreme Spirit are one and the

74

same. The difference lies in degree: the one is finite, the other infinite; the one is dependent, the other independent.

Ramakrishna

• Where should thou seek God? Seek Him in thy soul which is eternal in its nature and contains the divine birth.

Boehme

• Heaven is within thee. If thou seek God elsewhere, thou wilt never find Him.
Thou should not cry after God – the source is in thyself.

• I know that I have in me something without which nothing

could be. It is that I call God.

Angelus Silesius

• God cannot be recognised except in oneself. So long as thou findest Him not in thee, thou wilt not find Him anywhere. There is no God for the man who does not find Him in himself.

The greatest joy man can conceive is the joy of recognising in himself a being — free, intelligent, loving and in consequence happy, of feeling God in himself.

Man in order to be really a man must conceive the idea of God in himself.

Tolstoy

- While thou art saying 'I am alone with myself', in thy heart there is dwelling uninterruptedly that supreme spirit, silent observer of all good and all evil.

  Laws of Manu

- Thou seest Him, yet thou knowest not that thou seest.

  Thou are not, but only He.

  Thou art He and He is thou.

  All the attributes of Allah are thy attributes.

  Mohyuddin ibn Arabi

- The supreme Brahman, the self of all, the great abode of the universe, more subtle than the subtle, eternal, that is thyself and thou art that.

Kaivalya Upanishad

- Thou art that...not a part, not a mode of it, but identically that, the Absolute Spirit.

Chandogya Upanishad

- The essence of our being, the mystery in us which calls itself 'I', what words have we to express things like these? It is breath of heaven; the Highest reveals itself in man. This body, these faculties, this life that we live, is it not all a robe for Him who is nameless?

Carlyle

- God is myself; we are one in consciousness and His knowing is my knowing. If I were not, God would not be.

Eckhart

- The Purusha who is there and there, He am I.

Isha Upanishad

- They regarded the Divine Being and grew assured that it was no other than themselves...that they were themselves that Being...that they and that being made but one.

Farid-uddin Attar

Comments

The one and the only message coming from the teachers of diverse faiths and traditions is that the man or woman as soul is identical with God. This is the highest truth learnt on the spiritual path. There is a story in *Chandogya Upanishad* which says that initially there were two birds sitting on a tree full of alluring fruits. One of them was attracted by the fruits. It ate them and ran around to find more on different trees. Eventually it lost its identity. The other bird was not attracted by anything and so it retained its identity. The first bird is man and the second bird is God. The moment the first bird regains its original identity, it becomes God.

Practical Formulas for Jnana yoga

Listed below are practical formulas to make the path of knowledge easier to follow.

- Travel the path of pure reason leading to self-discovery.
- By ceaselessly asking the question 'Who am I'? one goes on removing cover after cover of ignorance.
- A stage comes when the mind ceases to exist and wisdom takes over.
- One realises immortality as the waking possession of the unborn and deathless self.

- Perceiving non-action while moving giant results opens the way to truth. In other words, believe, under all circumstances that you are not the doer, and remain free from the clutches of *karma*. Do good to others, but do not take pride in doing it.

- Concentrate on pain and find that it is a turning towards intense bliss and good. Pain teaches in three stages: endurance, equality of soul and ecstasy.

- Give up dependence on everything and everyone, become vulnerable, thus making room for God to enter you.

- One must either perfect renunciation of desires or perfect the satisfaction of desires. This leads to the truth, as in both cases desire perishes, which is the required precondition. Choose one of the ways and master it.

- Know that the inner renunciation of desire, ignorance and egoism, and not monasticism, is what leads one to truth. Thus by practising true renunciation one can become a *jnanayogi*. Acquiring knowledge and becoming a pundit is only the starting point.

- Whenever you come to know that *atma* and Brahman are identical, or that you and the father are one, know that you have known the truth.

Renunciation and Transcendence

Lord Krishna in the *Bhagavad Gita* advises that a person who is a true mystic is the one who is unattached to the fruits of his acts and who acts as he is obligated, not the person who lights no fire and performs no duty. Emphasis has been laid on the eight-fold yoga system, which helps in controlling the mind and the senses. People in general act with some self-interest or for some kind of self-gratification. Application of knowledge lies in acting in Krishna-consciousness and not for any kind of self-interest; such a person is said to be a true *sanyasi*.

Renunciation and yoga are one and the same thing, that is, linking oneself with the Lord — for one cannot become a *yogi* unless one renounces the desire for the satisfaction of the senses. A living entity is not independent but part of the Supreme. However, when one is entrapped in materialism, one becomes conditioned, while when one is in Krishna-consciousness, one is in one's real and natural form. Accordingly, the man of knowledge does not involve oneself in any kind of sense-gratification, rather he engages himself in yogic practices. However, a person living and acting in Krishna-consciousness is automatically a *sanyasi* and a *yogi*, at the same time. Such a person automatically fulfils the requirements of Jnana yoga. Giving up all activities for self-satisfaction and living only for the satisfaction of the Lord is the aim of the *jnanayogi*.

A person who is a beginner in the eight-fold yoga system, is supposed to use the means of work, while for a person who is already adept in yoga, the cessation of all material activity is the means. To link oneself to the Supreme, a person has to begin with the lowest material conditions and then arrive at the self-realised or spiritually elevated position. Although there are many ways or ladders of attaining this goal, the best way is through yoga, which has three divisions — Jnana yoga, Dhyan yoga and Bhakti yoga. A person who always thinks of the Lord, or in other words, one who is Krishna-conscious, from the beginning, is already on the level of meditation. Such a person is regarded as the one already out of material activities.

The purpose of the yoga system is to draw the mind away from the attachment of the objects of the senses. A beginner should try to deliver himself with the help of the mind, rather than degrade himself. The mind is both the friend of the conditioned soul as well as its enemy. The mind should be so trained that it can deliver the conditioned soul from the clutches of nescience. The soul is entangled in materialism because of the mind being attracted by the glitter of the material nature and associated desires for satisfaction of the senses. One can save the soul from the clutches of *maya*, not degrading oneself by the attraction of sense objects. The best way to do this is to engage oneself in Krishna-consciousness. A mind engaged in Krishna-consciousness becomes the cause of liberation. According to *Amrita-Bindu Upanishad,* "Mind is the cause of bondage and mind is the cause of liberation for man. Mind absorbed in sense objects is the cause of bondage, while the mind detached from sense objects is the cause of liberation."

One who has conquered the mind, has the mind as a best friend; while the one who has failed to do so, for him, his mind will remain the biggest enemy. The whole purpose of yoga is to control the mind and make it the best friend. The practice of yoga is a show and waste of time if the mind has not been controlled. Such an uncontrolled mind spoils the mission of life.

The unconquered mind takes one to the subordination of the five enemies – lust, greed, anger, attachment and ego. However, when the mind is conquered, one takes guidance from the Lord, who lives in the heart of everyone as Paramatma or Supersoul. The successful practice of yoga leads to the union of *atma* with Paramatma, that is, the soul with the Supersoul. And then, one gets directions directly from the Supersoul abiding in the heart.

For the person who has conquered mind, the Supersoul has already arrived, since he has attained tranquillity. Such a person finds happiness and distress, honour and dishonour to be the same. Since the mind has the habit of following dictation from some higher source, the following from the Paramatma automatically takes place as a transcendental property, and one is no more affected by the dualities of materialism. This is absorption in the

Supreme, and it is the practical form of *samadhi*.

One who establishes himself in such a self-realised position, is a *yogi* or a mystic. For such a person, everything — may it be pebbles, stones or gold — has the same value. One cannot understand the truth by bookish knowledge alone, unless one gets self-realisation personally. Only through transcendental service can one reach spiritual saturation, and then one can understand the form, quality and pastimes of the Lord. It is through transcendental knowledge that one can remain steady in his convictions, and not by the knowledge acquired through books, which can be misleading. Only the realised soul is self-controlled. Knowledge through books may be of golden value for others, but to a realised person it has no more value than pebbles or stones.

A *yogi* or transcendentalist should always engage his body, mind and self in relation to the Supreme; he should be living alone in a secluded place, and be always carefully controlling his mind. He should have freedom from desires and possessiveness. There are three different forms in which Absolute truth is realised — Brahman,

Paramatma and the supreme personality of the godhead. The impersonalists realise the Absolute as impersonal Brahman, the meditators realise Him as Paramatma or Supersoul sitting in everybody's heart, and a Krishna-conscious person realises Him as the personality of the godhead. Whatever one's belief or method of approach may be, one should be constantly engaged in one's particular pursuit, so that one can come to the highest perfection sooner or later. One should always keep one's mind on the highest goal, that is, the Supreme Lord. In other words, one should always think of Him and not forget Him even for a moment. Concentration of mind on the Lord is called trance or *samadhi*.

Living in a secluded place and avoiding being distracted by external objects, helps in concentration. One should be very careful in accepting conditions that are favourable to realisation, and rejecting those that are not favourable. One should also have a perfect determination with regard to material things, so that he/she does not hanker after them, which can persuade him/her to possess them.

An easy way to achieve all that is said above is to live and act in Krishna-consciousness. The right situation is to remain unattached to anything, and accept everything in relation to the Lord. Rejecting everything without the knowledge of its relationship to the Lord is not true renunciation. A Krishna-conscious person does not hanker for anything on his/her personal account because he/she is transcendental; but he/she accepts everything in relation to the Lord, since they all belong to Him.

For practising yoga, the practitioner should go to a secluded place and lay down on the ground *kusa grass* and cover it with deer skin and soft cloth. Care should be taken that the seat is neither too high nor too low, and that it is situated in a sacred place. The practitioner should then sit on it very firmly and practise yoga for the purification of the heart and the control of the mind, senses and activities, and then fix the mind at a single point. The sacred places in India are the places of pilgrimage, such as Mathura, Vrindavan, Rishikesh, Hardwar and Prayag; and places around sacred rivers, such as the Ganges and the Yamuna. Since all these conditions are not easy to be met with, the other way to achieve the goal of realisation is through chanting the holy name of the Lord. It is repeatedly emphasised that this is the only way and there is no other way.

The practitioner should hold one's body, neck and head in a straight line and stare steadily at the tip of the nose. In this way, having an unagitated and subdued mind, without fear and completely free from sex life, the practitioner should meditate upon Me with one's whole heart, and make Me the ultimate goal of one's life. The purpose of yogic practices is to realise the Lord sitting in the heart as Supersoul. One has to practise mind control and avoid all other kinds of sensual gratifications, of which sex life is the main factor. No one can perform the right type of yoga while indulging in sex. True celibacy means complete abstinence from sex in deed, words and mind, at all times, under all circumstances and in all places. In the real *ashrams*, therefore, celibacy is taught from early childhood, when one does not have even an inkling of what sex is. That is why children were sent to *gurukuls* at the age of five. However, a person having a regulated sex life with his/her own spouse only, is also accepted as a celibate, specially in

Bhakti yoga. This is so because devotion takes away the desire for sex gradually, and one finally becomes a real celibate. However, the paths of 'knowledge and concentration' do not allow sex at all because it is not eradicated, like it does, in the path of devotion. In Bhakti yoga one experiences superior taste, and so the desire for sex goes away automatically. But this does not happen in other paths. The aim of seeing the Lord within can thus be achieved.

A perverted memory keeps one fearful, because one has forgotten one's relationship with the Lord.

Living in Krishna-consciousness brings that memory back, and so the rules of yoga for Krishna-conscious people are slightly different. The path becomes easy and the goal appears approachable if one is used to live and act in Krishna-consciousness.

Practising constant control of the body, mind and activities, the *yogi*, having his/her mind regulated, attains the spiritual sky, by cessation of material existence. It is important to know that the spiritual sky, referred to here, is also known as *vaikunth*, 'kingdom of God' or the 'abode of the Lord.' One should clearly understand here that the aim of yoga is not just the improvement of health, but also cessation of all material existence. Simply aiming at the improvement of health through yoga, are not the symptoms of a *yogi*. The spiritual sky or the abode of the Lord is described in the *Bhagavad Gita* as the place which is self-illuminated — there is no sun, moon or electricity. The planets of the spiritual sky are the superior abodes and are also known as *paramdharma*. Through perfection of understanding, one can reach Lord Krishna's abode too, called 'Krishna-lok', where Krishna resides. The Lord in His abode, the all-pervading

Brahman, and the Paramatma or Supersoul—living in the hearts of everyone—are all synonymous statements. One realises the form of the Supreme Being according to one's belief. Thus, a person absorbed in Krishna-consciousness or a person who has perfected the yoga system, can overcome the path of birth and death and realise God.

Lord Krishna tells his beloved disciple Arjuna that a person who eats too much or eats too little, sleeps too much or does not sleep enough, cannot become a *yogi*. Similar advice came later from Gautam Buddha, who advocated the middle-way.

Buddha gave the example of a stringed musical instrument, which can produce a melodious sound only if the strings are neither too tight nor too loose. Lord Krishna prescribes the rule of regulated eating and sleeping for the practice of yoga. A person who eats more than necessary, will dream a lot and would sleep more than required. Unnecessary dreaming and excessive sleeping are both harmful for the person's regular and normal functioning. In fact, a sleep of six hours in the night is ideal, it is neither too much nor too little. According to medical reports, a sleep of one hour between 9 p.m. and 12 midnight is equal to two-and-a-half hours of normal sleep; a sleep of one hour between 12 midnight and 4 a.m. is equal to one-and-a-half hours of normal sleep; and a sleep of one hour after 4 a.m. is equal to only half-an-hour of normal sleep. My own experience over the years tells me that sleeping between 9 and 9.30 p.m. and getting up between 3 and 3.30 a.m. completes one's resting process and one feels fresh and energetic like a flower. And then, after washing oneself, one can sit down to chant mantras and meditate between 4 a.m. and 6 a.m., which is the best time for these practices. The spiritual forces in nature are awake at this time of the day, and one gets a natural enforcement of spiritual energy in oneself, if one chants and meditates at this time.

One who is regulated in one's habits of eating, sleeping, recreation and work, can practise yoga successfully, and thus reduce the severity of material pains. There are four normal requirements of the physical body eating, sleeping, mating and defending — which should be fulfilled. However, if one is careful, one can live in a regulated way in meeting these four demands, so that, everything is done in a balanced way, neither too much, nor too little. Such habits would eventually open the gateway of heaven, because, the individual would successfully perform yoga, and develop consciousness for the Lord. Something is always awake in a spiritually developed person. Even when sleeping, he is not really sleeping, while eating he is eating with the belief that the Lord is eating, while working he is working for the Lord, and his/her defending and mating demands are automatically adjusted to the minimum. Those who are living with Krishna-consciousness, for example, would do everything for the sake of Krishna and the upper and lower limits would adjust themselves automatically. Since the activities of such persons are untainted with personal interests and sense gratifications, the regulation takes place subconsciously and automatically. There is no material misery for such a person.

When the practitioner, by practising yoga, disciplines his mental activities and gets situated in transcendence, without any material desires, then he is said to be well-established in yoga. A *yogi* is known by the control he has on his mind, with regard to material desires, including sex. He cannot be disturbed by any kind of material desire. A Krishna-conscious person is supposed to be in such a situation, and he can be called a *yogi*.

Devotional services offered to the Lord can also lead to such a perfectional stage. The example of King Ambarish is very befitting in this context. He first engaged his mind on the pious feet of the Lord; then he engaged his words in describing the transcendental qualities of the Lord, one by one, his hands moving over the temple of the

Lord, his ears engaged in hearing of the activities of the Lord, his eyes searching the sight of the transcendental forms of the Lord, his body in touching the bodies of the other devotees, his nostrils trying to smell the scents of the lotus flowers decorating the lotus feet of the lord, his tongue trying to taste the *tulsi* leaves offered to the Lord, his legs moving to places where the Lord's various articles are at display and his head nodding to the tune of the respect paid to the Lord. Any devotee, who can engage himself like this fully into the Lord, deserves to be called a *yogi*. Such a transcendental stage is beyond description, and the impersonalists cannot understand it. One has to forget oneself and dissolve in the Lord, in all possible ways — the practitioner vanishes and the Lord remains, a situation known as *yukta* in the *Bhagavad Gita*.

A *yogi* or transcendentalist always remains steady in meditation and on his transcendent self, just as a lamp remains unwavering in a windless place. The characteristic of such a perfect state is that the practitioner is able to see his/her *atma* or self with a pure mind and relish and rejoice in it. One is situated in unbound transcendental happiness in that joyous state, which is realised through transcendental senses. Having established in this way, the practitioner never departs from the truth, and he believes that there is no greater gain than the one he has now. After being established in such a situation, the *yogi* is never shaken, even in the midst of greatest difficulties. This is really the actual freedom from the miseries of the material world. This is the yoga of the soul with the supersoul.

Sage Patanjali wrote the best treatise on yoga, some 2,600 years ago, which is more or less followed by everyone. However, a faster technique, based on modern research and personal experience, has been presented in the book on Hatha yoga, in the *All You Wanted to Know About* series. There are different schools of thought on the Patanjali system of yoga, where the resultant transcendental pleasure is accepted by some, and not accepted by others, because they want to maintain the theory of oneness. I would suggest that one should not fall into any kind of controversies, and follow the system of yoga that suits him/her the best. Requisite help will come to the practitioner from various sources, according to one's faith and devotion, from time to time. One will automatically pass from one stage of *samadhi* to another — *savikalpa* to *asampragyata* to *nirvikalpa*, when the eyebrow centre opens up and the experience of death (of ego) takes place. Truth is simple, but the theories make it complicated. Someone rightly said, "It is easier to become God than to know God." We are all gods in the making — what is needed is faith and sincerity.

The practitioner should engage himself/herself in the practice of yoga with faith and determination, and not stray from the path. One should remember that one has to master the means and not the end, since the end is bound to follow if the means are correctly applied. This much faith is essential.

Using intelligence sustained by full conviction, one should go into a trance gradually, and then the mind should be fixed on the self, without thinking of anything else. The fifth requirement of Patanjali's *Yoga sutra* is *pratyahar*, which means the cessation of sense activities. When the mind is thus engaged in thinking of the self, there is no danger of getting involved in materialistic conceptions. One good way of attaining such a state is by practising Krishna-consciousness.

Wherever the mind wanders, because of its flickering and unsteady nature, one must definitely put it back under the control of the self. The main purpose of yoga is to control the mind from its wandering nature. A self-realised *yogi* controls the mind and so he is called a *swami* or *goswami*. On the contrary, a person who is controlled by the mind, is said to be the servant of the senses and he is called *godasa*. A *swami* knows the art of directing his purified senses to the service of the Lord, and so he is said to be Krishna-conscious. Trying to remain always in Krishna-consciousness is one of the best ways of controlling the mind.

The Lord tells Arjuna that a *yogi* who has his mind fixed on Him verily attains the highest happiness. Such a practitioner is beyond the modes of passion; he is liberated through his qualitative identification with the Supreme, and is in this way, freed from all *karmic* reactions of the past. By fixing one's mind on the lotus feet of the Lord, one can remain in the quality of Brahman or the Absolute.

By constantly engaging oneself in the practice of yoga, the self-controlled *yogi* is freed from all material contamination, and achieves the highest stage of transcendental happiness. Knowing one's position in relation to the Lord, that is, to know that the soul is a part and parcel of the Supreme, is called self-realisation. This is the goal of Jnana yoga.

According to Lord Krishna, a true *yogi* sees Him in everyone and also sees everyone in Him.

He knows that everything is a manifestation of the Lord, nothing can exist without Him. At such a transcendental stage, which is beyond self-realisation, there develops an intimate relationship between the devotee and the Lord. Neither the living being can ever be annihilated, nor the Lord is ever out of the sight of the devotee. The same thing applies to the *yogi* who sees the Lord as Paramatma in the heart of everyone. Such a *yogi* becomes a pure devotee, who cannot bear to live without the Lord, even for a moment.

Such a *yogi*, who is engaged in the worshipful service of the Paramatma or Supersoul, knowing that he and the Supersoul are one, remains always in Him under all circumstances. During meditation on the Supersoul, the *yogi* may see the original form of Krishna, that is

Vishnu, from where He incarnated as *avatar*. The *yogi* should know that there is no difference between the different forms of the Lord and the forms of the Lord seen in various hearts. The very understanding that Lord Krishna is sitting in everybody's heart as the Supersoul, makes the *yogi* free from any faults. The *vedas* confirm that although the Lord is one, He is present in innumerable hearts. Similarly Vishnu is one, and yet He is all-pervading. Because of His inconceivable potency, in spite of His one form, He is present everywhere, just as the sun appears in many places at once.

One who sees the true equality of all beings, in both their happiness and their distress, by comparison to his own self, is a perfect *yogi*. A Krishna-conscious person is aware of everyone's happiness and distress, in comparison to himself, and hence, he can be called a perfect *yogi*. This is a lesson for the *jnanayogi*.

Perfection in Yoga

Arjuna expressed his doubt to Lord Krishna that the system of yoga, which He has summarised, appears impractical and unendurable to him, because the mind remains restless and unsteady. People are engaged in a bitter struggle for living. There is little possibility that they would be able to observe the strict rules laid down by the yoga system. For example, though Arjuna was favourably endowed in many ways, regulating the mode of living, the manner of sitting, choosing an appropriate place and detaching the mind from material thoughts was not so easy. Arjuna belonged to the kingly race and was a warrior having very good health,and above all, he was a personal friend of Lord Krishna. If he found it impractical in that age, how can it possibly be practical in the present times? Those who are able to observe the rules of yoga and accomplish it, must be exceptionally good people.

Arjuna says that the mind is restless, turbulent, obstinate and very strong, and according to him, it is more difficult to control the mind than to control the wind. The mind is supposed to be subservient to intelligence, but in reality it is so strong and obstinate that intelligence finds itself unable to control the mind.

According to *Katha Upanishad*, "The material body is a cart in which the individual is a passenger and intelligence is the driver.

The mind is the driving instrument and the senses are the horses pulling the cart. The self, in association with the mind and senses, is either the enjoyer or the sufferer, according to the situation. This is what the great thinkers understand." Accordingly, the mind is supposed to obey the intelligence, but the former is so strong that it overtakes its own intelligence. It is only through yoga that such a strong mind can be controlled, and for people these days, performance of yoga is not so easy.

It was later found by the great practitioners that the chanting of *mantras* is the right means of controlling the mind. I can say this with my own experience that chanting a *mantra* for longer periods of time daily, is really the effective measure for subduing the mind. During the first hour of chanting the mind keeps wandering; during the second hour it is semi-controlled; and during the third hour it completely forgets the phenomenal world and the practitioner is likely to reach the altered state of consciousness. The duration of time between two chantings goes on increasing, and it is this in-between space which brings connection to the altered state of consciousness.

Lord Krishna agrees with Arjuna and admits that it is really very difficult to curb the restless mind; however, it is possible to do so with detachment and regular practice. There are always some people who are able to observe the strict rules of yoga, although with some moderation here and there, and achieve the goal of self-realisation. Nevertheless, there is an easier though longer and safer method of developing Krishna-consciousness. This method consists of devotional practices, beginning with hearing about Krishna. One gradually transcends thoughts about the phenomenal world, and gets the mind detached from activities that are not devoted to the Lord. This eventually leads to *vairagya* or renunciation of the material world. Those who find it difficult to concentrate on the impersonal aspect of God may find it easier to do so on Krishna's activities. The more one hears about Krishna in different ways, the more one gets closer to the Supreme Spirit, experiencing spiritual satisfaction. Just as food gives satisfaction to the body, so hearing the names of Krishna and engaging in activities connected with Him gives satisfaction to the inner self. It is just like curing a disease with medicines. Hearing of the transcendental activities of Lord Krishna and eating the blessed food, which has first been offered to the Lord, is an expert treatment for the obstinate mind, which is otherwise hard to control. This is the process of Krishna-consciousness.

An individual, whose mind is unbridled, would find self-realisation to be difficult. However, one whose mind is controlled and one who strives using appropriate methods, will surely succeed. This is the opinion of Lord Krishna. Practicing yoga without controlling the mind would be a waste of time. Practicing yoga and being fully immersed in the material world are opposing activities. It may not lead to spiritual realisation. It is therefore necessary to control the mind through devotional practices, and then perform yoga simultaneously. This is combining Bhakti yoga with

Hatha yoga and is the ideal combination. In fact, the path of Integral yoga, which combines Hatha yoga, Jnana yoga, Bhakti yoga and Tantra yoga, is the shortest method of all to arrive at the goal of self-realisation.

Arjuna asked the Lord about the destination of unsuccessful practitioners, who began the process of self-realisation with faith, but later were diverted due to interest in the material world, and thus could not complete the process of mysticism. Knowing the truth means the understanding that one is not the body and mind, but the permanent entity called soul or *atma*. This understanding can be attained by Jnana yoga or Bhakti yoga or by other methods, such as the eight-fold path of Patanjali. By whatever method one may reach the goal, it leads to transcendental bliss and knowledge. In Chapter 2 of the *Bhagavad Gita* the Lord has confirmed this. However, since the methods are difficult and time consuming, and the means of perfection are at times not available or one may get attracted to something in the material world, one may not be able to complete the process in a single lifetime. Despite constant endeavour one may fail in one's attempt. It is like declaring war on the illusory *maya*. Arjuna wants to know the fate of such people who for one reason or the other could not complete the process of self-realisation.

Arjuna expresses his doubt about such people who are distracted from the path of transcendence, and fall away from both spiritual and material success and perish, with no position in any walk of life. Pythagoras drew a figure with two opposing offshoots, meaning thereby that either a person can progress in the material world or in the spiritual path, but not in both at the same time.

Other spiritual leaders of different faiths have said the same thing. On the material path one may acquire wealth, position, power and so on. On the spiritual path one sacrifices all material goals in favour of bliss and knowledge. Arjuna's doubt concerns people who, while in the middle of the spiritual path, get deviated to the material path; consequently they may loose both the worlds. The material world they would have already renounced, while the spiritual world is not theirs either, due to distraction while in it. What should be the destiny of such people?

Arjuna requests Krishna to dispel his doubt completely. He further says that it is only He, and no one else, who can destroy his doubt. Since philosophers and sages are still at the mercy of the material world, they are not capable of clearing Arjuna's doubt. Lord Krishna being the knower of the past, present and future of all living entities, is the only right person who can answer his question.

Lord Krishna replies that a transcendentalist engaged in auspicious activities does not get destroyed either in this world or in the spiritual world. One who does good can never be overcome by evil. For an individual who gives up the material world and takes refuge in the Lord, needs to fear no loss or degradation for him or her in any way. However, a non-devotee may fully engage in professional duties and yet may not be able to gain anything. An individual on the spiritual path may not have completed the requirements of the prescribed duties, yet he may not be a looser, since engaging oneself in Krishna-consciousness is very auspicious and its account is never lost. Even if such a person is born into a family of low status in the next life, he or she continues to remain on the path of Krishna-consciousness. On the other hand, an individual who may strictly follow the prescribed duties without being engaged in Krishna-consciousness is not likely to attain the auspicious result.

Human beings can be divided into two clear categories — regulated and unregulated. Those who confine themselves to the four basic requirements of eating, sleeping, defending and mating, remain always in the material existence. Such people may be civilised or uncivilised, educated or uneducated, strong or weak, yet they have no auspicious gain at all. These are the unregulated people. On the other hand, there are people who follow the prescribed duties of the scriptures and gradually make progress on the path of Krishna-consciousness. Such people are said to be regulated, and even if they are unable to complete the mystical process, they do make progress in life.

There are classifications of the people who are engaged in auspicious activities too. Firstly, there are people who enjoy material prosperity, together with following the rules and regulations of the scriptures. Secondly, there are people whose aim is to find liberation from *maya*. Thirdly, there are people who are engaged purely in Krishna-consciousness. The people of the first category can be further divided into two classes — those who expect the fruits of their labour, and those who do not expect the fruits of their labour. The ones with expectation of the fruits of labour can be promoted to a better life on this planet or may go to another higher planet; yet they are not following the right path, which is auspicious. This is because they have not been able to renounce the fruits of their labour. The only right path therefore is the one in

139

which people are engaged in Krishna-consciousness. Any path which does not totally converge on liberation and self-realisation alone is left with some blemishes, which will not let one achieve the final goal. All the austerities of life suffered on the path of Krishna-consciousness will pay their dividend in the end. Since the eight-fold path of yoga also takes one finally to Krishna-consciousness, the direct path of Krishna- consciousness is the right one.

An unsuccessful *yogi* enjoys for many, many years on the planets where pious entities are living, and then he or she is born into a family of righteous people, or into a family, which is rich and aristocratic. There are two categories of *yogis* who have fallen from the path — firstly, the ones who fall after very little progress and secondly, the ones who fall after a long practice of yoga. The practitioners of the first category proceed to higher planets where pious living entities are permitted. Individuals live there for a pretty long time and in this they learn a lot of good things, which prepare them eventually for birth into a family with righteous or aristocratically rich people. All this is preparation for achieving Krishna- consciousness, after the individual gets material satisfaction and purification by living with people of the right kind. Birth into a rich and aristocratic family is designed by nature for the soul to take advantage of the facilities and to elevate oneself to the higher levels in Krishna- consciousness.

A *yogi* who has failed after a long practice of yoga takes birth in a family of transcendentalists who are recognised for the great wisdom they possess. Definitely, a birth of this kind is not a common thing. A soul born into a family of spiritual perfectionists is certainly rare, and it provides an early advantage to the young child on the path to self-realisation. Such children are likely to become spiritual masters in their lifetime, providing help to other younger souls. Although famous families such as the 'acharya' and 'goswami' families do not commonly exist now, but there are still such families, which foster true spiritualists from one generation to another. Accordingly, it is lucky to be born into one such family and complete the process of self-realisation.

I know about my own previous life in which I was a *yogi* but I could not complete the process. In this life

I got the opportunity to be born into a family of spiritualists. I got an early introduction to the chanting of *mantras* and its relevance from my maternal grandfather. Later I obtained a doctorate in mathematics and served as a professor in eight countries. In the teaching profession I had plenty of time to devote to yoga, meditation, reading of the scriptures and joining various spiritual and metaphysical bodies all over the world. I could easily devote about six hours every day to these pursuits, after fulfilling my responsibilities in mathematics. After experiencing *kundalini* I resigned from my job in

1994, and thereafter affluent people in the USA supported me financially so that I could carry on my pursuits. Certainly all this has been the grace of the Lord and help from nature. I know of others too who had similar experiences.

Getting such a birth, the individual revives Divine consciousness from his or her previous incarnation and proceeds from there onwards to achieve completeness. A very good example in this context is King Bharata, after whose name India was known as Bharata-Varsa. He began following the spiritual path early, but was not successful. In his next life he was born into a family of learned *Brahmans*. However, he had the habit of not talking to anyone and remaining secluded, and so he was nick-named as Jada Bharata (*jada* means inert as a root). King Rahugana later discovered him to be one of the greatest transcendentalist. The life of Bharata illustrates the fact that the practice of yoga never goes waste, it is credited to one's account which can be cashed at any point of time. At other places one can find sayings that indicate that spiritual progress is always credited to one's account, even if one gets diverted to materialism. Whenever one way or the other revives it, one proceeds from there onwards. It is a linear progression; the soul always proceeds from where it left off in some incarnation, without losing whatever was gained. The grace of the Lord always helps and provides opportunities to the practitioner to achieve perfection on the spiritual path. Several examples can be quoted in this regard.

By virtue of the Divine consciousness from a previous incarnation, one automatically gets attracted to the principles of yoga, even without seeking them. Such an inquisitive transcendentalist can always be seen above mere rituals described in the scriptures. Ordinary or middle-order practitioners are seen entangled in the age-old rituals of various faiths and traditions, and they acquire bookish knowledge only. *Yogis* of the higher order, on the other hand, go directly to advanced yogic practices leading to transcendental experiences, and complete the process of self-realisation in that lifetime. I know some of my own relatives, who are older than me, and even after three to four hours of ritualistic practices in the early hours of the morning during their whole life, have not risen above bookish knowledge. They could not get a single direct experience, although they talk well on the basis of their education, studies and orthodox practices. One could clearly see the difference between such people and those who have had transcendental experiences. One who has seen the truth, and whose questions have been answered, talks with such confidence about facts related to the beyond, which others cannot do.

The *Vedas* talk about people who chant the holy names of God with love and devotion, and say that such people have already crossed the orthodox barriers of rituals, sacrifices, austerities, bathing in sacred places and studying the scriptures. Even if such souls are born into different religions, such as the famous poet Rahim and Thakur Haridasa born into Muslim families, their love and power of chanting holy names cannot remain hidden for long. These people plunge directly into God-consciousness by chanting, without wasting time in mechanical rituals. Certainly, they must have passed through the formalities of sacrifices and austerities in previous incarnation(s), which normally is the prerequisite to chanting the names of the Lord.

When the *yogi* engages himself with sincere effort to make further progress, having cleared himself of all kinds of contamination, then in the end, acquiring completion after several births of practice, one attains the final goal, that is, Krishna-consciousness. Once born into a rich and aristocratic family, the soul finds all kinds of comfort and facilities to complete his or her unfinished journey towards spiritual perfection. He or she then begins with sincere efforts, getting oneself cleaned of all contamination, and reaches the highest level of Krishna-consciousness. According to Chapter 7, verse 28 of the *Bhagavad Gita*, "After many, many births of performing pious activities, when one attains complete freedom from all contaminations, and from all kinds of illusory dualities, one engages oneself in the transcendental loving service of the Lord."

Lord Krishna tells Arjuna that a *yogi* is greater than an ascetic, greater than the empiricist and greater than the fruitive worker. Therefore, under all circumstances, one should try to become a *yogi*. Yoga being the direct link between the soul and the

Supersoul, a *yogi* is said to be greater than all kinds of practitioners. However, there have been different yogic approaches to the same goal. Thus, the path of selfless action is called Karma yoga, the path of knowledge is called Jnana yoga and the path of devotion is called Bhakti yoga. Then there is the path of physical posture and austerities called Hatha yoga, and the path that recognises the sex drive is called Tantra yoga. Lord Krishna only mentions that the approach of yoga is better than other approaches; he does not say which kind of yoga is to be followed. However, the three

Vedas, that is the *Rig-Veda, Yajur-Veda* and *Sama-Veda* talk about the three basic yogas — Karma yoga, Jnana yoga and Bhakti yoga, respectively. At one place Lord Krishna says that in the *Vedas* He is *Sama-Veda,* which is the exponent of Bhakti yoga. From this, one can infer that He likes the path of devotion to be the best among others, that is, Bhakti yoga is the highest form of yoga. In fact, Karma yoga brings equanimity in the practitioner, Jnana yoga brings the knowledge of the existence of God, and then Bhakti yoga brings the realisation of God with bliss and inner happiness. From this one may

154

infer that the path of devotion is finally the best way to God. This is gradually made clear by the Lord in His further sayings which are as follows:

Amongst all the *yogis*, the one who always abides in Me with great faith, thinks of Me within himself, and renders transcendental loving service to Me, he is the one united most intimately with Me in yoga and he is the highest of all.

The Lord makes it quite clear that it is not the usual kind of worship which He is referring to. Worship usually means to adore, to show respect and honour to someone who is worthy of it. One may worship even a benevolent political leader, or a social reformer or redeemer. But this is not the meaning here. He means love, devotion and service to the Lord with single-mindedness. According to *Shrimad-Bhagavatam*, "A person who does not render service and neglects his duty to the primeval Lord, who is the source of all living beings, he/she will certainly fall down from his/her constitutional position."

Seeing all this one may conclude that all kinds of yoga practices finally culminate into Bhakti yoga, that is, the path of devotion. One may further infer from this that whenever Lord Krishna talks about yoga, He means Bhakti yoga or the path of devotion. It is a different matter that one may have to pass through other kinds of yogas to successfully arrive at Bhakti yoga in the end. Sri Aurobindo has also touched this point when he says that Jnana yoga provides one with the understanding that there is a Supreme power in the universe, but it does not give the taste of it. The path of selfless action or Karma yoga is the beginning of the path. While engaged in Karma yoga the practitioner begins to gain knowledge and is lead to renunciation. This is the beginning of Jnana yoga. The path of knowledge or Jnana yoga leads to dry knowledge of God, there is no enjoyment at heart or the feeling of bliss inside. While engaged in Jnana yoga, the practitioner increases his or her meditation with attention on the Supreme, and reaches the stage of Ashtanga yoga. When the practice of Ashtanga yoga crosses a certain level, the practitioner comes closer to the Lord, which is the end of all yoga. This is devotion to God or Bhakti yoga, and this is after one has come to know about His existence. So the right way for the *yogi* is to pass through all other *yogic* systems that have been mentioned earlier, and gradually transcending them one after another, he should finally arrive at Bhakti yoga. It is here that the practitioner realises oneness with God and proclaims '*Aham Brahmasmi*' or 'I Am That I Am.'

There is nothing more to do now. There is no practice left behind. He/she has merged with the Supreme.

Other titles in the series

- Bhakti Yoga

- Karma Yoga

- Hatha Yoga

- Kriya Yoga

- Kundalini

- Mantras

- Aura

- Dreams

- Tantra Yoga

- Psychic Development

- Chakras and Nadis